CONTENTS

1
INTRODUCTIONS

Depression and anxiety are different conditions, but they commonly occur together. They also have similar treatments.

Feeling down or having the blues now and then is normal. And everyone feels anxious from time to time — it's a normal response to stressful situations. But severe or ongoing feelings of depression and anxiety can be a sign of an underlying mental health disorder.

Anxiety may occur as a symptom of clinical (major) depression. It's also common to have depression that's triggered by an anxiety disorder, such as generalized anxiety disorder, panic disorder or separation anxiety disorder. Many people have a diagnosis of both an anxiety disorder and clinical depression.

Symptoms of both conditions usually improve with psychological counseling (psychotherapy), medications, such as antidepressants, or both. Lifestyle changes, such as improving sleep habits, increasing social support, using stress-reduction techniques or getting regular exercise, also may help. If you have either condition, avoid alcohol, smoking and recreational drugs. They can make both conditions worse and interfere with treatment.

CHAPTER 1
. RECOGNIZING WHY

Anxiety and depression can have many different causes, and often result from a combination of factors. Here are some common factors that can contribute to the development of anxiety or depression:

1. Genetics: Studies have shown that there is a genetic component to anxiety and depression. If someone in your family has experienced anxiety or depression, you may be at an increased risk.

2. Environmental factors: Certain environmental factors, such as stress at work, financial problems, or a traumatic event, can trigger anxiety or depression.

3. Brain chemistry: Chemical imbalances in the brain can contribute to anxiety and depression. For example, imbalances in the levels of serotonin, dopamine, and norepinephrine have all been linked to these conditions.

4. Personality: Some personality traits, such as being highly self-critical or having a negative outlook on life, can make a person more prone to anxiety and depression.

5. Medical conditions: Certain medical conditions, such as thyroid disorders or chronic pain, can increase the risk of anxiety and depression.

6. Substance abuse: Substance abuse can both contribute to and result from anxiety and depression.

It's important to note that everyone's experience with anxiety and depression is unique, and there may be additional factors that contribute to these conditions. If you are struggling with anxiety or depression, it's important to seek professional help to get a proper diagnosis and treatment plan tailored to your individual needs

CHAPTER 2
KNOW YOUR TRIGGERS

Identifying the triggers of anxiety can be a complex process, as different people may have different triggers and it may not always be clear what is causing the anxiety. Here are some strategies that may be helpful in identifying your own triggers:

1. Keep a journal: Write down your thoughts, feelings, and physical sensations when you experience anxiety. Over time, you may start to notice patterns or common themes that could be triggers.

2. Reflect on past experiences: Think about times when you have felt anxious in the past. What was happening at the time? What were you thinking or feeling? This may help you identify triggers that you were not previously aware of.

3. Talk to a therapist: A mental health professional can help you identify triggers and develop coping strategies. They can also provide a safe and supportive environment for exploring your emotions and experiences.

4. Take note of your physical symptoms: Anxiety can often manifest in physical symptoms such as a racing heart, sweating, or trembling. Keeping track of these symptoms can help you identify triggers that may be causing them.

5. Pay attention to your thoughts: Notice any negative or anxious thoughts that pop into your head throughout the day. Identifying and challenging these thoughts can help reduce anxiety and uncover triggers.

Remember that identifying triggers is just one step in managing anxiety. It's important to also develop coping strategies and seek professional help if needed.

CHAPTER 3
COPING MECHANISM

Coping mechanisms can be helpful in managing anxiety and reducing its impact on daily life. Here are some coping strategies that may be useful:

1. Deep breathing: Practice deep breathing exercises to help calm your mind and reduce physical symptoms of anxiety.

2. Mindfulness meditation: Mindfulness meditation involves focusing on the present moment without judgment. It can be helpful in reducing anxiety and increasing feelings of relaxation.

3. Exercise: Regular exercise can help reduce anxiety and improve mood. Find an activity that you enjoy and make it a regular part of your routine.

4. Progressive muscle relaxation: This technique involves tensing and then relaxing different muscle groups in the body. It can help reduce physical tension and promote relaxation.

5. Cognitive-behavioral therapy: CBT is a type of therapy that can help you identify and change negative thought patterns and behaviors that contribute to anxiety.

6. Connect with others: Talking to friends, family members, or a mental health professional can provide a supportive environment for managing anxiety.

7. Get enough sleep: Adequate sleep is important for mental and physical health. Try to establish a consistent sleep schedule and create a relaxing bedtime routine.

Remember that coping mechanisms may be different for everyone, and it may take some trial and error to find what works best for you. It's also important to seek professional help if your anxiety is significantly impacting your daily life.

CHAPTER 4
PRACTICING DEEP BREATHING

Deep breathing can be a helpful technique for managing anxiety. When you feel anxious, your body enters into a "fight or flight" response, which can cause rapid breathing and a feeling of shortness of breath. By practicing deep breathing exercises, you can slow down your breathing and activate your body's relaxation response.

Here's how to practice deep breathing for anxiety:

1. Find a quiet, comfortable place to sit or lie down.

2. Close your eyes and focus your attention on your breath.

3. Inhale slowly and deeply through your nose, filling your lungs with air.

4. Hold your breath for a few seconds.

5. Exhale slowly and fully through your mouth, releasing all the air from your lungs.

6. Repeat this cycle for several minutes, focusing on your breath and allowing your body to relax.

There are several different types of deep breathing exercises that you can try. One popular technique is the 4-7-8 breathing exercise, which involves inhaling for a count of four, holding for a count of seven, and exhaling for a count of eight.

Deep breathing can be a helpful technique for managing anxiety because it helps to slow down your breathing and activate your body's relaxation response. It can also be practiced anywhere, at any time, making it a convenient tool for managing anxiety in the moment.

However, it's important to note that deep breathing alone may not be enough to treat anxiety in the long term. It is often most effective when combined with other coping strategies, such as therapy or medication.

CHAPTER5
MINDFULNESS

Mindfulness is a technique that involves paying attention to the present moment with a non-judgmental and accepting attitude. Practicing mindfulness can be helpful in reducing anxiety and improving overall well-being.

Here are some ways that mindfulness can help with anxiety:

1. Reducing negative thinking: Mindfulness can help you become more aware of negative or anxious thoughts, and develop a more accepting and non-judgmental attitude towards them. This can help reduce their impact on your mental and emotional state.

2. Improving emotional regulation: By practicing mindfulness, you can become more aware of your emotional state and learn to regulate it more effectively. This can help reduce the intensity and duration of anxiety symptoms.

3. Increasing resilience: Mindfulness can help you develop greater resilience to stress and adversity, allowing you to bounce back more easily from difficult situations.

4. Enhancing relaxation: Mindfulness can promote relaxation and reduce physical tension, which can help reduce symptoms of anxiety.

There are many different ways to practice mindfulness, including meditation, deep breathing, and body scan exercises. One simple mindfulness exercise is to focus on your breath and bring your attention back to it whenever your mind wanders. Over time, you can gradually increase the amount of time you spend practicing mindfulness and incorporate it into your daily routine.

CHAPTER 6
EXERCISE AND MOVEMENT

Exercise and movement can be helpful in managing anxiety by reducing stress and improving overall physical and mental health.

Here are some ways that exercise and movement can contribute to the treatment of anxiety:

1. Reducing stress: Exercise can help reduce stress by releasing endorphins, which are natural chemicals that promote feelings of well-being and reduce the perception of pain. Regular exercise can also help regulate cortisol, a hormone associated with stress.

2. Promoting relaxation: Exercise can promote relaxation by reducing muscle tension and increasing body awareness. This can help reduce physical symptoms of anxiety, such as rapid heartbeat and shortness of breath.

3. Improving mood: Exercise has been shown to improve mood by increasing levels of neurotransmitters such as serotonin and dopamine, which are associated with feelings of happiness and well-being.

4. Boosting confidence: Regular exercise can help improve self-esteem and confidence, which can be especially helpful for individuals with anxiety.

5. Providing a distraction: Exercise can provide a healthy distraction from anxious thoughts and worries, allowing individuals to focus on the present moment and engage in a positive activity.

There are many different types of exercise and movement that can be helpful for managing anxiety, including yoga, running, swimming, and dance. It's important to find an activity that you enjoy and that fits your individual needs and preferences.

If you're new to exercise, it's important to start slowly and gradually increase the intensity and duration of your workouts. Consult with a healthcare professional before starting any new exercise program, especially if you have any underlying medical conditions or concerns.

SPECIFIC EXERCISES THAT HELPS IN IMPROVEMENT OF ANXIETY

There are specific types of exercise and movement that have been shown to be particularly effective in managing anxiety. Here are some examples:

1. Aerobic exercise: Aerobic exercise, such as running, cycling, or swimming, can be effective in reducing anxiety symptoms.

This type of exercise releases endorphins, which can help promote feelings of well-being and reduce stress.

2. Yoga: Yoga combines physical postures with breathing techniques and meditation, making it a holistic practice that can help reduce anxiety symptoms. Yoga has been shown to be effective in reducing stress and improving overall mental and physical health.

3. Tai chi
Tai chi is a gentle, low-impact exercise that originated in China as a martial art. It involves a series of slow, flowing movements that are performed in a mindful and relaxed manner, accompanied by deep breathing and mental focus. Tai chi is often described as a moving meditation, and has been shown to have numerous benefits for physical and mental health, including reducing anxiety symptoms.

Here are some ways that tai chi can help with anxiety:

1. Promoting relaxation: The slow, flowing movements of tai chi can help reduce muscle tension and promote relaxation, which can help reduce physical symptoms of anxiety such as rapid heartbeat and shallow breathing.

2. Improving focus: Tai chi involves focusing the mind on the present moment and the movements of the body, which can help reduce anxious thoughts and worries.

3. Reducing stress: Tai chi has been shown to reduce levels of cortisol, a hormone associated with stress, and increase levels of endorphins, which can promote feelings of well-being and reduce pain.

4. Improving balance and coordination: Tai chi can help improve balance and coordination, which can be especially beneficial for older adults who may be at risk for falls or injuries.

5. Enhancing overall health: Tai chi has been shown to have numerous benefits for overall physical and mental health, including improving flexibility, reducing chronic pain, and improving sleep quality.

If you're interested in trying tai chi, you can look for classes or instructional videos online. It's important to start slowly and gradually increase the intensity and duration of your practice.

For patients who may not have the physical strength to undergo tai chi exercises, there are alternative exercises that can also be helpful in managing anxiety. Here are some examples:

1. Chair exercises: Chair exercises can be a good alternative for patients who may not have the physical strength or mobility to perform standing exercises. These exercises can be done while seated in a chair, and can include movements such as arm raises, leg extensions, and seated twists.

2. Breathing exercises: Breathing exercises, such as deep breathing, can be helpful in reducing anxiety symptoms by promoting relaxation and reducing stress. These exercises can be done anywhere, at any time, and involve taking slow, deep breaths in through the nose and out through the mouth.

3. Mindfulness meditation: Mindfulness meditation involves focusing the mind on the present moment and cultivating a non-judgmental awareness of thoughts, feelings, and bodily sensations. This practice can help reduce anxious thoughts and worries, and promote feelings of calm and relaxation.

4. Gentle stretching: Gentle stretching exercises, such as yoga poses modified for chair use, can be helpful in reducing muscle tension and promoting relaxation. These exercises can be done while seated in a chair or lying down on a mat.

It's important to consult with a healthcare professional before starting any new exercise program, especially if you have any underlying medical conditions or concerns. They can help you determine which exercises and movements are safe and appropriate for your individual needs and abilities.

CHAPTER 7
RELAXATIONS

Relaxation techniques can be an effective tool in the treatment of anxiety disorders. Anxiety can lead to physical symptoms such as increased heart rate, rapid breathing, and muscle tension. Relaxation techniques can help to counteract these symptoms by calming the body and promoting a sense of relaxation and calmness. Here are some of the benefits of relaxation in the treatment of anxiety:

1. Reducing Physical Tension: When we feel anxious, our muscles tend to tighten up, leading to physical tension and discomfort. Relaxation techniques such as progressive muscle relaxation or yoga can help to release this tension, resulting in a decrease in physical symptoms of anxiety.

2. Lowering Heart Rate and Blood Pressure: Anxiety can cause an increase in heart rate and blood pressure, which can be damaging to the body over time. Relaxation techniques such as deep breathing or meditation can help to lower these physiological responses, reducing the risk of heart disease and other related conditions.

3. Promoting Calmness and Mental Clarity: When we feel anxious, our thoughts can become jumbled and unclear, making it difficult to focus or make decisions. Relaxation techniques can help to promote mental clarity and a sense of

calmness, allowing us to think more clearly and make better decisions.

4. Improving Sleep: Anxiety can make it difficult to fall asleep or stay asleep, leading to fatigue and a decrease in overall quality of life. Relaxation techniques such as guided imagery or progressive muscle relaxation can help to promote better sleep, leading to increased energy and a greater sense of well-being.

5. Enhancing Overall Well-Being: When we feel relaxed and calm, we are better able to enjoy life and engage in activities that promote our overall well-being. Relaxation techniques can help to reduce the impact of anxiety on our daily lives, allowing us to live more fully and joyfully.

It is important to note that relaxation techniques alone may not be enough to treat severe anxiety disorders, and should be used in conjunction with other forms of therapy or medication as necessary. However, incorporating relaxation techniques into a comprehensive treatment plan can be a valuable tool in managing symptoms and promoting overall well-being.

Chapter 8

WAYS TO IMPROVE WORK RELATED ANXIETY
Certainly,There are some ways to improve work-related anxiety:

1. Identify the root cause: Try to identify the specific cause or trigger of your anxiety at work. This could be a particular task, coworker, or deadline. Once you have identified the source of your anxiety, you can develop strategies to manage it.

2. Practice relaxation techniques: Incorporate relaxation techniques such as deep breathing, mindfulness meditation, or yoga into your daily routine. These techniques can help you manage stress and anxiety at work.

3. Set boundaries: It's important to set boundaries to prevent work from taking over your personal life. This could include setting specific work hours or taking breaks throughout the day.

4. Prioritize self-care: Make sure to prioritize self-care activities such as exercise, eating well, and getting enough sleep. Taking care of your physical health can have a positive impact on your mental health.

5. Seek support: Talk to someone you trust, such as a friend, family member, or therapist, about your work-related anxiety.

Having a support system can help you manage your anxiety and provide perspective.

6. Develop coping skills: Learn coping skills that work for you, such as positive self-talk or visualization techniques. These skills can help you manage anxiety in the moment.

7. Consider therapy or counseling: If your work-related anxiety is severe, consider seeking professional help. A therapist or counselor can work with you to develop a plan to manage your anxiety and improve your mental health.

WAYS IN WHICH PETS CAN HELP TO IMPROVE ANXIETY

Here are some ways that pets can help improve anxiety and depression:

1. Companionship: Pets provide unconditional love and companionship, which can help alleviate feelings of loneliness and isolation that can contribute to anxiety and depression.

2. Stress relief: Petting or playing with a pet can release endorphins and lower cortisol levels, which can help reduce stress and anxiety.

3. Routine and responsibility: Caring for a pet provides a sense of routine and responsibility, which can be especially helpful for those struggling with depression. Having a pet that

relies on you for their care can also provide a sense of purpose and meaning.

4. Exercise and outdoor time: Many pets, such as dogs, require daily exercise and outdoor time. This can encourage their owners to get outside and move their bodies, which can help improve mood and decrease anxiety.

5. Mindfulness and presence: Pets can help their owners stay present in the moment and practice mindfulness. Focusing on playing with or caring for a pet can help quiet the mind and reduce anxious or depressive thoughts.

6. Social interaction: Owning a pet can also provide opportunities for social interaction, such as walking a dog in the park or chatting with other pet owners. This can help reduce feelings of loneliness and increase social support.

7. Unconditional love and acceptance: Perhaps most importantly, pets offer unconditional love and acceptance. This can be especially powerful for those struggling with anxiety or depression, who may feel that they are unworthy of love or struggle to form connections with others.

For those who have pet allergies, there are still alternatives that can help improve anxiety and depression:

1. Plant care: Taking care of plants can provide many of the same benefits as caring for a pet, such as routine,

responsibility, and mindfulness. Many people find that tending to their plants and watching them grow can be very therapeutic.

2. Virtual pets: There are many apps and websites that offer virtual pet companions that can provide a sense of companionship and routine. While they may not offer the same physical interaction as a real pet, they can still provide a sense of comfort and purpose.

3. Animal-assisted therapy: Animal-assisted therapy is a type of therapy that involves interactions with trained therapy animals, such as dogs or horses. The animals are carefully selected for their temperament and trained to provide comfort and support to individuals with a range of mental health conditions.

4. Outdoor activities: Spending time in nature and participating in outdoor activities, such as hiking or gardening, can provide many of the same benefits as owning a pet. Getting outside and moving your body can help reduce stress and improve mood.

5. Creative activities: Engaging in creative activities, such as painting, writing, or playing music, can be a great way to reduce anxiety and depression. These activities can provide a sense of purpose and allow individuals to express themselves in a way that feels meaningful.

It's important to remember that everyone's mental health journey is different, and what works for one person may not work for another. struggling with anxiety or depression, it's important to talk to a healthcare professional who can help you develop a personalized treatment plan.

FOOD AND SUPPLEMENTS THAT HELPS IN TREATMENT OF ANXIETY

here are some supplements and foods that may help in the treatment of anxiety and depression:

1. Omega-3 fatty acids: Omega-3s can be found in fatty fish such as salmon, mackerel, and sardines, as well as in supplements. Studies have shown that omega-3 fatty acids may help reduce symptoms of depression and anxiety.

2. Magnesium: Magnesium is an important mineral that plays a role in many bodily functions, including the regulation of mood. Foods that are high in magnesium include spinach, almonds, avocados, and black beans.

3. Probiotics: There is emerging evidence that suggests that gut health may play a role in the development and treatment of mental health disorders. Probiotics, which are beneficial bacteria that live in our gut, may help improve mood and reduce symptoms of anxiety and depression. Probiotic-rich foods include yogurt, kefir, sauerkraut, and kimchi.

4. Vitamin D: Vitamin D is important for overall health and well-being, and studies have shown that it may play a role in the development and treatment of depression. Vitamin D can be found in fatty fish, egg yolks, and fortified foods like milk and cereal.

5. B vitamins: B vitamins, particularly vitamin B12 and folate, play a role in the production of neurotransmitters that are involved in mood regulation. Foods that are high in B vitamins include leafy greens, legumes, and fortified cereals.

It's important to note that while these supplements and foods may be helpful for some people with anxiety and depression, they are not a substitute for professional treatment.

Ashwagandha is a popular herb used in traditional Ayurvedic medicine to promote physical and mental health. Ashwagandha gummies, which are made from the root of the ashwagandha plant, are a convenient way to consume this herb. Here are some potential benefits of ashwagandha gummies:

1. May help reduce stress and anxiety: Ashwagandha has been shown to have anxiolytic (anti-anxiety) effects in some studies. Some research has also suggested that ashwagandha may help lower cortisol levels, a hormone that is released in response to stress.

2. May help improve mood: Ashwagandha has been shown to have mood-boosting effects in some studies. It may help improve symptoms of depression and anxiety, which can also improve overall mood.

3. May help improve sleep: Ashwagandha has been shown to have sedative effects in some studies, which may help improve

sleep quality. Better sleep can also help improve mood and reduce stress.

4. May help boost cognitive function: Some research suggests that ashwagandha may help improve cognitive function, including memory and attention.

5. May help reduce inflammation: Ashwagandha has been shown to have anti-inflammatory effects in some studies. Chronic inflammation has been linked to a number of health problems, including depression and anxiety.

Note that ashwagandha gummies may have these potential benefits, they are not a substitute for professional medical advice or treatment., it's important to speak with a mental health professional.

There are several other herbs and roots that have been studied for their potential benefits in the treatment of depression and anxiety. Here are a few examples:

1. Rhodiola rosea: Rhodiola is an adaptogenic herb that has been shown to have antidepressant and anxiolytic effects in some studies. It may help improve mood, reduce fatigue, and improve cognitive function.

2. St. John's wort: St. John's wort is a plant that has been used for centuries to treat a variety of ailments, including depression. Some studies have suggested that it may be as

effective as antidepressant medication for mild to moderate depression.

3. Kava: Kava is a plant native to the South Pacific that has been used for its calming effects. It may help reduce anxiety and promote relaxation, but it should be used with caution as it can interact with some medications and may have potential side effects.

4. Passionflower: Passionflower is a plant that has been used to treat anxiety and insomnia. It may help reduce anxiety and promote relaxation without causing drowsiness.

5. Valerian root: Valerian is a root that has been used to treat anxiety and insomnia. It may help reduce anxiety and improve sleep quality.

Other natural food and fruits that can help are:

1. Blueberries: Blueberries are high in antioxidants, which can help protect the brain from oxidative stress, which has been linked to depression and anxiety.

2. Salmon: Salmon is a great source of omega-3 fatty acids, which have been shown to have antidepressant effects.

3. Dark chocolate: Dark chocolate contains compounds such as flavonoids, which may have mood-enhancing effects.

4. Spinach: Spinach is high in magnesium, which has been linked to reduced symptoms of depression.

5. Avocado: Avocado is a good source of healthy fats and vitamin E, which may help improve mood and reduce anxiety.

6. Almonds: Almonds are high in magnesium, zinc, and healthy fats, which may help reduce symptoms of anxiety and depression.

7. Berries: Berries are high in vitamin C, which has been shown to help reduce symptoms of depression.

8. Turmeric: Turmeric contains a compound called curcumin, which has been shown to have antidepressant effects.

9. Greek yogurt: Greek yogurt is high in probiotics, which may help improve mood and reduce anxiety.

10. Chamomile tea: Chamomile tea is a natural calming agent that may help reduce symptoms of anxiety and promote relaxation.

Remember you're not alone there are millions of people out here fighting the same battle, Better days are coming you have been through alot, it's time to shine.
Don't hesistate to:

1. Seek professional help: Depression is a serious mental health condition that can be difficult to manage on your own.

It's important to seek the help of a mental health professional who can provide you with the support and treatment you need.

2. Practice self-care: Self-care is essential for managing depression. This may include getting enough sleep, eating a balanced diet, exercising regularly, and engaging in activities that bring you joy.

3. Challenge negative thoughts: Depression can cause negative thinking patterns that can worsen symptoms. It's important to challenge these negative thoughts and replace them with positive ones.

4. Stay connected: Isolation can worsen symptoms of depression. It's important to stay connected with friends and family, even if it's through virtual means.

5. Set realistic goals: Setting small, achievable goals can help you feel more accomplished and boost your mood.

6. Be patient and kind to yourself: Recovery from depression is a process that takes time. It's important to be patient and kind to yourself as you navigate this journey.

7. Consider joining a support group: Connecting with others who are going through similar experiences can be helpful in managing depression.

Remember, recovery from depression is possible with the right treatment and support. Don't be afraid to reach out for help and remember to take care of yourself along the way.

NOTES